I. Introduction

In a world increasingly reliant on synthetic medications and technological advancements, there's a growing yearning for a return to nature, a rediscovery of ancient healing wisdom that has sustained humanity for millennia. "The Complete Guide to Medicinal Herbs: Harnessing Nature's Healing Power emerges as a beacon guiding modern seekers back to the roots of healing, illuminating the profound therapeutic potential found within the embrace of nature's pharmacy.

In this comprehensive guide, we embark on a journey through the rich tapestry of medicinal herbs, traversing the annals of history, culture, and science to unveil the profound significance and enduring relevance of herbal medicine. As we delve into the healing wisdom of medicinal herbs, we are invited to rediscover a holistic approach to health and well-being, one that honors the interconnectedness of mind, body, and spirit.

The allure of medicinal herbs lies not only in their therapeutic properties but also in their deep-rooted history, spanning ancient civilizations and diverse cultures across the globe. From the revered healing practices of ancient Egypt and Greece to the intricate herbal traditions of China and India, the use of medicinal herbs has been woven into the fabric of human existence, offering remedies for ailments and insights into the mysteries of life itself.

Yet, as we stand on the precipice of the modern age, the significance of medicinal herbs remains as potent as ever, resonating with a growing movement towards holistic health and natural living. In a world fraught with the complexities of modern medicine and environmental degradation, the resurgence of interest in herbal medicine represents a return to simplicity, a rekindling of our innate connection to the earth and its bountiful offerings.

Within the pages of this guide, readers will embark on a transformative journey of discovery, exploring the myriad benefits and applications of medicinal herbs for health, healing, and vitality. From immune-boosting tonics and stress-relieving teas to soothing salves and revitalizing tinctures, each chapter serves as a gateway to unlocking the healing potential of nature's botanical treasures.

Moreover, "The Complete Guide to Medicinal Herbs" transcends mere instruction, embodying a philosophy rooted in reverence for the natural world and a commitment to sustainable living. As stewards of the earth, we are called to cultivate a deeper relationship with the plants that nourish and heal us, fostering a symbiotic partnership that honors the delicate balance of life.

As we embark on this journey together, let us embrace the wisdom of ancient healers and modern pioneers alike, weaving a tapestry of healing that honors the timeless tradition of herbal medicine while embracing the possibilities of the future. Through the collective wisdom of generations past and present, we discover the transformative power of medicinal herbs, illuminating a path towards holistic health, vitality, and harmony with the natural world.

A. The History and Significance of Medicinal Herbs

In the intricate tapestry of human history, there exists a thread that has endured through the ages, weaving its way through ancient civilizations, medieval monasteries, and modern societies alike. This thread is none other than the profound significance of medicinal herbs, a treasure trove of healing wisdom that has stood the test of time.

The story of medicinal herbs is as ancient as humanity itself, stretching back to the dawn of civilization when our ancestors first walked the earth. In the cradle of ancient civilizations such as Egypt, Mesopotamia, and China, herbal medicine flourished as a cornerstone of healing practices. The Ebers Papyrus, an ancient Egyptian medical text dating back to around 1550 BCE, contains references to over 700 medicinal plants, highlighting the advanced knowledge of herbal remedies in ancient societies.

The Greeks, too, contributed significantly to the development of herbal medicine, with renowned figures such as Hippocrates and Dioscorides documenting the medicinal properties of various plants. Hippocrates, often referred to as the father of modern medicine, famously proclaimed, "Let food be thy medicine and medicine be thy food," emphasizing the importance of natural remedies in maintaining health and preventing disease.

In the medieval era, herbal medicine continued to thrive, with monasteries serving as centers of herbal knowledge and experimentation. Monastic herbalists meticulously cataloged and cultivated medicinal herbs, preserving ancient wisdom while expanding upon it through empirical observation and trial-and-error.

One such luminary of medieval herbalism was Hildegard von Bingen, a German Benedictine abbess and polymath who penned several works on herbal medicine, including "Physical" and "Causae et Curae." Hildegard's holistic approach to healing emphasized the interconnectedness of body, mind, and spirit, laying the groundwork for modern herbal medicine.

The Age of Exploration brought about a new chapter in the history of medicinal herbs, as European explorers traversed the globe in search of new botanical treasures. Plants such as ginseng from Asia and cinchona bark from South America found their way into European pharmacopeias, leading to the development of important herbal remedies for various ailments.

As the scientific revolution unfolded, herbal medicine faced increasing scrutiny and skepticism from proponents of modern medicine. However, the resurgence of interest in natural remedies in the 20th century paved the way for a renaissance in herbal medicine, as researchers began to explore the pharmacological properties of medicinal plants with renewed vigor.

Today, the significance of medicinal herbs extends far beyond historical curiosity, resonating deeply with a global movement towards holistic health and sustainable living. In an era marked by the overuse of synthetic medications and the depletion of natural resources, the allure of herbal medicine lies in its gentle yet potent approach to healing, rooted in the wisdom of nature.

From immune-boosting herbs and stress-relieving adaptogens to soothing botanicals for skin care and digestive health, the therapeutic potential of medicinal herbs is vast and diverse. Moreover, the cultivation and preservation of medicinal herbs offer a sustainable alternative to conventional pharmaceuticals, promoting environmental stewardship and biodiversity conservation.

In conclusion, the history and significance of medicinal herbs serve as a testament to the enduring relationship between humanity and the natural world. Across cultures and centuries, the healing wisdom of medicinal herbs has transcended boundaries, offering solace, sustenance, and hope to generations past, present, and future. As we continue to navigate the complexities of modern life, let us not forget the timeless wisdom of herbal medicine, a beacon of healing light amidst the tumultuous seas of change.

B. Understanding the Healing Properties of Plants

In an age where modern medicine dominates the healthcare landscape, there's a growing recognition of the profound healing potential found within the natural world. From the lush rainforests of the Amazon to the sun-drenched fields of Provence, plants have long been revered for their ability to alleviate ailments, soothe the soul, and restore balance to the body. As we delve deeper into the intricate web of phytochemicals and bioactive compounds found within these botanical wonders, we uncover a treasure trove of therapeutic properties that have been honed by millions of years of evolution.

At the heart of plant-based healing lies a diverse array of compounds, each with its unique set of medicinal properties. Take, for example, the vibrant hues of turmeric, which owe their color to curcumin, a potent anti-inflammatory compound renowned for its ability to reduce pain and inflammation. Similarly, the delicate blossoms of chamomile contain chamazulene and apigenin, compounds that impart soothing and anti-anxiety effects, making it a popular choice for promoting relaxation and sleep.

Yet, the healing properties of plants extend far beyond their individual constituents, encompassing a holistic approach to health and well-being that addresses the interconnectedness of mind, body, and spirit. In traditional medicine systems such as Ayurveda and Traditional Chinese Medicine (TCM), plants are revered not only for their physical benefits but also for their ability to restore harmony and balance to the entire being.

Take, for instance, the practice of forest bathing, a Japanese tradition that involves immersing oneself in the sights, sounds, and aromas of the forest to promote relaxation and reduce stress. Scientific research has shown that spending time in nature can lower cortisol levels, decrease blood pressure, and boost mood, highlighting the therapeutic benefits of simply being in the presence of plants.

Moreover, plants offer a wealth of benefits for mental and emotional well-being, nurturing the spirit and uplifting the soul. The delicate fragrance of lavender, for instance, has been shown to reduce anxiety and improve sleep quality, while the bright blooms of sunflowers evoke feelings of joy and optimism. In a world marked by stress and uncertainty, the healing power of plants offers a sanctuary of solace and renewal, reminding us of our deep-rooted connection to the natural world.

In recent years, scientific research has begun to unravel the mechanisms underlying the healing properties of plants, shedding light on their potential applications in modern medicine. From the development of novel herbal remedies to the synthesis of plant-derived pharmaceuticals, the field of botanical medicine is experiencing a renaissance, fueled by a growing recognition of the limitations of conventional pharmaceuticals and the desire for more natural, sustainable alternatives.

However, as we harness the healing power of plants, it's essential to approach their use with respect, reverence, and a deep understanding of their ecological and cultural significance. Sustainable harvesting practices, ethical wildcrafting, and the preservation of biodiversity are crucial considerations in ensuring the long-term viability of plant-based healing traditions.

In conclusion, the healing power of plants offers a timeless and holistic approach to health and well-being that resonates with the rhythms of nature itself. From the forests to the fields, the botanical treasures of the earth stand as a testament to the resilience, adaptability, and generosity of the natural world. By honoring and harnessing nature's pharmacy, we embark on a journey of healing and transformation that transcends boundaries, uniting us in our shared quest for health, vitality, and harmony with the earth.

C. Why Herbal Medicine is Gaining Popularity

In an era dominated by technological advancements and pharmaceutical innovations, there's a growing movement towards embracing the wisdom of nature and returning to traditional healing practices. Herbal medicine, once relegated to the fringes of mainstream healthcare, is experiencing a resurgence in popularity as people seek natural alternatives to conventional treatments. From herbal teas and tinctures to botanical supplements and remedies, the allure of herbal medicine lies in its holistic approach to health and well-being, addressing not only the symptoms of illness but also the underlying imbalances within the body.

One of the primary reasons for the growing popularity of herbal medicine is a growing disillusionment with the limitations and side effects of conventional pharmaceuticals. While pharmaceutical drugs can be highly effective in treating specific symptoms, they often come with a host of potential side effects and risks. Many people are turning to herbal medicine as a gentler, more sustainable alternative, one that works in harmony with the body's natural healing mechanisms rather than against them.

Moreover, herbal medicine offers a more personalized approach to healthcare, with remedies tailored to individual needs and preferences.

Unlike one-size-fits-all pharmaceuticals, herbal remedies can be customized to address a wide range of health concerns, from digestive issues and immune support to stress relief and sleep disturbances. This personalized approach resonates with many people who are seeking more autonomy and control over their health.

Another driving force behind the popularity of herbal medicine is a growing recognition of the importance of holistic health and wellness. In today's fast-paced world, many people are seeking ways to reconnect with nature and cultivate a deeper sense of balance and harmony in their lives. Herbal medicine offers a pathway to holistic healing, addressing not only physical symptoms but also the mental, emotional, and spiritual aspects of well-being.

Furthermore, the resurgence of interest in herbal medicine is fueled by a desire for sustainability and environmental stewardship. As concerns about the ecological impact of pharmaceutical manufacturing and over-reliance on synthetic chemicals grow, many people are turning to herbal remedies as a more eco-friendly and sustainable option. By harnessing the healing power of plants, we can reduce our dependence on fossil fuels, minimize pollution, and support biodiversity conservation.

Additionally, the democratization of information through the internet and social media has played a significant role in popularizing herbal medicine. With a wealth of online resources, blogs, and social media influencers sharing information about herbal remedies and natural health practices, people have unprecedented access to knowledge about herbal medicine and its benefits. This accessibility has empowered individuals to take charge of their health and explore alternative healing modalities.

In conclusion, the growing popularity of herbal medicine reflects a broader cultural shift towards embracing natural, holistic approaches to health and wellness. As people seek alternatives to conventional pharmaceuticals and strive for greater sustainability and balance in their lives, herbal medicine offers a compelling solution. By harnessing the wisdom of nature and embracing the healing power of plants, we can embark on a journey of holistic healing and well-being that honors the interconnectedness of all living beings.

II. Getting Started with Medicinal Herbs

A. Embrace Curiosity and Openness:

The first step in getting started with medicinal herbs is to approach the process with an open mind and a spirit of curiosity. Allow yourself to be guided by intuition and a sense of wonder as you explore the vast and diverse world of herbal medicine. Remember that herbal healing is as much an art as it is a science, and there is no one-size-fits-all approach. Be willing to experiment, learn from your experiences, and trust in the wisdom of nature.

2. Educate Yourself:

Before diving headfirst into the world of medicinal herbs, take some time to educate yourself about the basics. Familiarize yourself with common medicinal herbs, their properties, and their traditional uses. There are countless books, online resources, and herbal courses available to help you deepen your understanding of herbal medicine. Consider joining local herbalism groups or attending workshops and seminars to connect with experienced herbalists and learn from their wisdom.

3. Start Small:

When it comes to experimenting with medicinal herbs, it's best to start small and gradually expand your repertoire as you gain confidence and experience. Choose a few herbs that resonate with you or address specific health concerns you'd like to support. Focus on building a strong foundation of knowledge and experience with these herbs before branching out to explore others. Some beginner-friendly herbs to consider include chamomile for relaxation, peppermint for digestion, and lavender for stress relief.

4. Choose Quality Herbs:

When purchasing medicinal herbs, it's important to choose high-quality, organic herbs from reputable sources. Look for herbs that have been ethically harvested and processed to ensure their potency and purity. If possible, consider growing your own herbs in a garden or indoor planter to have a fresh supply on hand whenever you need them. Remember that the quality of the herbs you use will directly impact their effectiveness, so it's worth investing in the best quality you can afford.

5. Experiment with Different Preparations:

Medicinal herbs can be prepared and consumed in a variety of forms, including teas, tinctures, capsules, salves, and poultices. Experiment with different preparations to find what works best for you and your unique needs. Keep a journal to track your experiences with different herbs and preparations, noting any changes in symptoms or overall well-being. Don't be afraid to get creative and explore new ways of incorporating herbs into your daily routine.

6. Trust Your Intuition:

As you embark on your journey with medicinal herbs, remember to trust your intuition and listen to your body's wisdom. Pay attention to how different herbs make you feel and honor your body's signals and sensations. If something doesn't feel right or doesn't resonate with you, don't force it – there are plenty of other herbs and remedies to explore. Trust that your body knows what it needs and be gentle with yourself as you navigate the healing process.

A. Basics of Herbal Medicine

1. Understanding the Principles:

Herbal medicine is based on the principle that plants contain bioactive compounds with medicinal properties that can promote health and alleviate illness. These compounds may include alkaloids, flavonoids, terpenes, and essential oils, among others. Herbalists draw upon this rich

pharmacopeia

of plant constituents to formulate remedies that address a wide range of health concerns.

2.Holistic Approach:

Unlike conventional medicine, which often focuses on treating isolated symptoms or diseases, herbal medicine takes a holistic approach to health and wellness. Practitioners of herbal medicine view the body as a dynamic ecosystem, where physical, mental, emotional, and spiritual factors are interconnected and influence one another. Herbal remedies are chosen not only for their specific therapeutic actions but also for their ability to restore balance and harmony to the entire being.

3.Herbal Actions and Properties:

Medicinal herbs exhibit a variety of therapeutic actions and properties, each with its unique effects on the body. Some herbs are known for their anti-inflammatory properties, which can help reduce pain and swelling, while others have antimicrobial properties that can combat infections. Additionally, herbs may be classified according to their energetics, such as warming or cooling, moistening or drying, which can further inform their therapeutic use.

4.Preparation and Administration:

Medicinal herbs can be prepared and administered in a variety of forms, including teas, tinctures, capsules, salves, poultices, and essential oils. The choice of preparation depends on the specific properties of the herb, as well as the desired therapeutic effect and individual preferences. Herbalists may also recommend dietary and lifestyle modifications to complement herbal treatment and support overall health.

5.Safety and Precautions:

While herbal medicine is generally considered safe when used appropriately, it's essential to exercise caution and consult with a qualified healthcare practitioner before using medicinal herbs, especially if you have underlying health conditions, are pregnant or breastfeeding, or are taking medications. Some herbs may interact with medications or have contraindications for certain populations, so it's essential to seek personalized guidance to ensure safe and effective treatment.

6.Cultivating a Relationship with Plants:

At its heart, herbal medicine is about cultivating a deep connection with the natural world and honoring the wisdom of plants. Spending time in nature, observing plant life cycles, and learning to identify medicinal herbs in their natural habitats can deepen your understanding and appreciation of herbal medicine. By fostering a relationship with plants, you can tap into their healing energy and gain insight into their therapeutic potential.

B. Tools and Equipment Needed

When preparing medicinal herbs, having the right tools and equipment is essential to ensure that you can effectively extract the therapeutic properties of the plants and create high-quality herbal remedies. Here are some essential tools and equipment needed for preparing medicinal herbs:

- 1. Mortar and Pestle: A mortar and pestle are traditional tools used for grinding and pulverizing dried herbs. This manual method helps release the active compounds within the herbs, allowing for better extraction during preparation.
- 2. Herb Grinder: An herb grinder is a convenient alternative to a mortar and pestle, especially for grinding larger quantities of herbs quickly and efficiently. Herb grinders come in various sizes and designs, including manual and electric models.
- 3.Herb Scissors or Knife: Sharp herb scissors or a knife are essential for cutting and chopping fresh herbs before use. This allows for precise preparation and ensures that the herbs are properly processed for extraction.

- 4.Strainer or Cheesecloth: A fine-mesh strainer or cheesecloth is used to strain herbal infusions, decoctions, and tinctures, separating the liquid from the solid plant material. This ensures a smooth and clear final product.
- 5.Glass Jars and Bottles: Glass jars and bottles are ideal for storing herbal preparations such as tinctures, infused oils, and herbal vinegars. Glass is non-reactive and helps preserve the potency and freshness of the herbs.
- 6.Double Boiler or Crockpot: A double boiler or crockpot is used for gently heating herbs in carrier oils to create infused oils and salves. This indirect heating method prevents the herbs from overheating and ensures a gradual extraction of their therapeutic properties.

- 7.Kitchen Scale: A kitchen scale is helpful for accurately measuring dried herbs and other ingredients when preparing herbal remedies. This ensures consistency and precision in the formulation of herbal preparations.

- 8. Measuring Cups and Spoons: Measuring cups and spoons are essential for accurately measuring liquid ingredients such as water, alcohol, and carrier oils when preparing herbal infusions, tinctures, and other remedies.
- 9. Funnel: A funnel is useful for transferring herbal preparations into storage containers without spilling or wasting any liquid. Choose a funnel with a wide mouth to accommodate various bottle sizes.

- 10. Labels and Markers: Labels and markers are essential for clearly labeling herbal preparations with their names, ingredients, and preparation dates. This helps you keep track of your remedies and ensures safe and proper usage.

By having these essential tools and equipment on hand, you can confidently prepare medicinal herbs and create a variety of herbal remedies to support health and well-being. Whether you're making herbal teas, tinctures, salves, or infused oils, having the right tools ensures that you can effectively extract and preserve the therapeutic properties of the plants for optimal healing results.

C. Safety Precautions and Considerations

1. Research and Education: Before using any medicinal herb, take the time to research its properties, potential side effects, and contraindications. Familiarize yourself with reputable sources of information, such as herbal books, websites, and healthcare practitioners

1. Consultation with Healthcare Practitioner: If you have underlying health conditions, are pregnant or breastfeeding, or are taking medications, consult with a qualified healthcare

practitioner before using medicinal herbs. Some herbs may interact with medications or have contraindications for certain populations, so it's essential to seek personalized guidance to ensure safe and effective treatment.

1. Start with Small Doses: When trying a new herb for the first time, start with a small dose and gradually increase it as needed. This allows you to assess your tolerance and sensitivity to the herb and reduces the risk of adverse reactions.
2. Allergies and Sensitivities: Be mindful of potential allergies or sensitivities to certain herbs. If you have known allergies to plants in the same botanical family or have experienced allergic reactions to herbs in the past, exercise caution and avoid using those herbs.

1. Quality and Purity: Choose high-quality, organic herbs from reputable sources to ensure their potency and purity. Avoid herbs that have been sprayed with pesticides or other chemicals, as these may contain harmful residues that can compromise their safety and efficacy.

1. Proper Dosage and Administration: Follow recommended dosage guidelines for each herb and preparation method. Take care to administer herbal remedies according to instructions to avoid overconsumption or misuse. If unsure, consult with a qualified herbalist or healthcare practitioner for guidance.

1. Monitor for Adverse Effects: Pay attention to how your body responds to herbal remedies and monitor for any adverse effects or allergic reactions. Discontinue use and seek medical attention if you experience symptoms such as nausea, vomiting, rash, difficulty breathing, or dizziness.

1. Interactions with Medications: Be aware of potential interactions between medicinal herbs and medications you may be taking. Some herbs can enhance or inhibit the effects of

certain medications, leading to unwanted side effects or reduced efficacy. Always inform your healthcare provider about any herbal supplements you are using to prevent potential interactions.

1. Storage and Handling: Store medicinal herbs in a cool, dry place away from direct sunlight and moisture to maintain their potency and freshness. Use airtight containers to prevent contamination and degradation of the herbs over time.

1. Respect for Nature and Sustainability: Practice ethical wildcrafting or source herbs from sustainable suppliers to support biodiversity conservation and minimize environmental respect for Nature and Sustainability: Practice ethical wildcrafting or source herbs from sustainable suppliers to support biodiversity conservation and impact. Harvest herbs responsibly and avoid overharvesting or depleting wild population

By following these safety precautions and considerations, you can use medicinal herbs responsibly and enjoy their therapeutic benefits while minimizing the risk of adverse

effects. Remember to approach herbal medicine with respect, reverence, and a commitment to your health and well-being.

III. Herbal Remedies for Common Ailments

A. Herbal Remedies for Immune Support

1. Echinacea (Echinacea purpurea):

- Echinacea is one of the most well-known herbs for immune system support. It contains compounds such as polysaccharides and alkamides that stimulate the activity of white blood cells and enhance the body's natural defense mechanisms against infections.

- Echinacea can be taken in various forms, including capsules, tinctures, teas, and extracts. It's often used at the onset of cold or flu symptoms to help shorten the duration and severity of illness.

2. Astragalus (Astragalus membranaceus):

- Astragalus is a powerful adaptogenic herb that helps strengthen the immune system and increase resistance to stress and illness. It contains polysaccharides and flavonoids that support immune cell function and enhance immune response.
- Astragalus is commonly used in traditional Chinese medicine to support immune health and prevent respiratory infections. It can be taken as a tea, tincture, or capsule for long-term immune support.

3. Elderberry (Sambucus nigra):

- Elderberry is rich in antioxidants, vitamins, and flavonoids that help boost the immune system and reduce inflammation. It has antiviral properties that can help prevent and alleviate symptoms of colds and flu.
- Elderberry syrup is a popular remedy for immune support, especially during cold and flu season. It can also be taken in the form of capsules, teas, or lozenges.

4.Garlic (Allium sativum):

- Garlic is a potent antimicrobial herb that has been used for centuries to support immune health and fight infections. It

contains allicin, a sulfur compound with antibacterial, antiviral, and antifungal properties.
- Raw garlic is most effective for immune support, but it can also be taken in the form of capsules, tinctures, or added to food for its immune-boosting benefits.

5.Ginger (Zingiber officinale):

- Ginger is a warming herb that helps stimulate circulation and support immune function. It has anti-inflammatory and antimicrobial properties that can help prevent and alleviate symptoms of respiratory infections.
- Ginger can be taken as a tea, added to soups and stir-fries, or consumed in the form of capsules or tinctures for immune support.

6.Reishi Mushroom (Ganoderma lucidum):

- Reishi mushroom is a powerful adaptogenic herb that helps modulate the immune system and increase resistance to stress. It contains polysaccharides and triterpenes that support immune cell activity and enhance immune response.
- Reishi mushroom can be taken as a tea, tincture, or powder for immune support. It's often used in traditional Chinese medicine to strengthen the body's defenses and promote overall well-being.

These herbal remedies can be incorporated into your daily routine to support immune system health and resilience. However, it's essential to consult with a healthcare practitioner before starting any new herbal regimen, especially if you have underlying health conditions or are taking medications. Additionally, remember to prioritize overall wellness practices such as proper nutrition, adequate sleep, regular exercise, and stress management to optimize immune function.

2. Recipes for Immune-Boosting Teas and Tonics

- Ginger Lemon Immunity Tea:

- 1-inch piece of fresh ginger, sliced
- 1 tablespoon fresh lemon juice
- 1 teaspoon raw honey (optional)
- 2 cups of water

Instructions:

- Bring water to a boil in a saucepan.
- Add ginger slices to the boiling water and simmer for 5-10 minutes.
- Remove from heat and stir in lemon juice and honey (if using).
- Strain into cups and enjoy. Drink this tea regularly to support your immune system.

Turmeric Immunity Tonic:

- 1 teaspoon ground turmeric
- 1 teaspoon raw honey
- 1/2 teaspoon ground cinnamon
- Pinch of ground black pepper (to enhance turmeric absorption)
- 1 cup of hot water
- Optional: a slice of fresh ginger or a squeeze of lemon juice

Instructions:

- Add turmeric, honey, cinnamon, black pepper, and any optional ingredients to a mug.
- Pour hot water over the ingredients and stir well until everything is dissolved.
- Let it steep for a few minutes, then sip slowly. Enjoy this tonic regularly to support your immune system.

Echinacea Elderberry Immune-Boosting Tea:

- 1 tablespoon dried echinacea root or 1 echinacea tea bag
- 1 tablespoon dried elderberries or 1 elderberry tea bag
- 1 teaspoon dried rose hips
- 1 teaspoon dried thyme
- 2 cups of water
- Optional: raw honey to taste

Instructions:

- In a saucepan, bring water to a boil.
- Add echinacea root, elderberries, rose hips, and thyme to the boiling water.
- Reduce heat and simmer for 10-15 minutes.
- Strain the tea into cups and add honey to taste if desired. Sip on this immune-boosting tea regularly during cold and flu season.

Garlic Honey Immunity Tonic:

- 3-4 cloves of garlic, minced
- 1 tablespoon raw honey
- Juice of 1/2 lemon
- Optional: a pinch of cayenne pepper

Instructions:

- Mix minced garlic, honey, lemon juice, and cayenne pepper (if using) in a small bowl.
- Let the mixture sit for at least 30 minutes to allow the flavors to meld.
- Consume 1 teaspoon of this tonic daily to support immune function. You can take it straight or mix it with warm water.

Remember to consult with a healthcare professional before incorporating new herbal remedies into your routine, especially if you have any underlying health conditions or are pregnant or breastfeeding. These teas and tonics can complement a healthy lifestyle but should not replace medical treatment if you are ill.

B. Digestive Health

1. Herbs for Digestive Issues

1. Peppermint: Peppermint is known for its soothing properties on the digestive system. It can help relieve symptoms of indigestion, such as bloating, gas, and stomach cramps. Peppermint tea or capsules are commonly used.

1. Ginger: Ginger is another well-known herb for digestive issues. It helps to stimulate digestion, reduce nausea, and alleviate stomach discomfort. You can consume ginger tea, ginger capsules, or simply add fresh ginger to your meals.

1. Chamomile: Chamomile has anti-inflammatory properties and can help soothe the stomach lining. It is commonly used to relieve symptoms of indigestion, such as gas and bloating. Chamomile tea is a popular way to consume this herb.

1. Fennel: Fennel seeds are often used to relieve symptoms of bloating, gas, and indigestion. They can be chewed after meals or brewed into a tea.

1. Licorice root: Licorice root can help soothe the stomach lining and reduce inflammation. It is often used to treat conditions like acid reflux and heartburn. However, it's important to use deglycyrrhizinated licorice (DGL) for digestive issues, as regular licorice can cause side effects when used long-term.

1. Turmeric: Turmeric contains a compound called curcumin, which has anti-inflammatory properties. It can help alleviate symptoms of inflammatory bowel diseases like Crohn's disease and ulcerative colitis. Turmeric can be consumed in capsule form or added to food.

1. Slippery elm: Slippery elm is a demulcent herb that can help soothe and protect the digestive tract. It is often used to relieve symptoms of heartburn, gastritis, and ulcers. Slippery elm is typically consumed as a powder mixed with water.

1. Marshmallow root: Like slippery elm, marshmallow root is a demulcent herb that can help soothe and protect the digestive tract. It is often used to relieve symptoms of heartburn, gastritis, and ulcers. Marshmallow root can be consumed as a tea or taken in capsule form.

1. Artichoke leaf: Artichoke leaf extract can help improve digestion by increasing bile production and reducing symptoms of indigestion, such as bloating and gas. It is commonly consumed in capsule form.

1. Lemon balm: Lemon balm has carminative properties, meaning it can help relieve gas and bloating. It is often used to aid digestion and reduce symptoms of indigestion. Lemon balm tea is a popular way to consume this herb.

Before using any herbal remedies for digestive ailments, it's important to consult with a healthcare professional, especially if you have any underlying health conditions or are taking medications, as some herbs may interact with certain medications or may not be suitable for everyone. Additionally, herbal remedies should not be used as a substitute for medical treatment for serious digestive issues.

2. DIY Herbal Digestive Remedies

Ginger Tea: Peel and slice fresh ginger root, then simmer it in water for about 10 minutes to make ginger tea. You can add honey and lemon for flavor. Ginger tea aids digestion, relieves nausea, and reduces bloating.

Peppermint Tea: Steep fresh or dried peppermint leaves in hot water for peppermint tea. Peppermint tea helps relax the muscles of the digestive tract, relieving symptoms of indigestion, gas, and bloating.

Fennel Seed Infusion: Crush fennel seeds and steep them in hot water for 10-15 minutes. Strain and drink tea. Fennel seed infusion can help relieve gas, bloating, and indigestion.

Chamomile Tea: Steep chamomile flowers in hot water for chamomile tea. Chamomile tea has anti-inflammatory properties and can help soothe the stomach, reducing symptoms of indigestion and bloating.

Turmeric Milk: Mix turmeric powder with warm milk and a dash of black pepper. Turmeric milk has anti-inflammatory properties and can help soothe the digestive system.

Lemon Balm Tea: Steep lemon balm leaves in hot water for lemon balm tea. Lemon balm tea has carminative properties, which can help relieve gas and bloating.

Dandelion Root Tea: Roast and grind dandelion roots, then steep them in hot water for dandelion root tea. Dandelion root tea stimulates digestion and can help relieve constipation and bloating.

Licorice Root Decoction: Simmer licorice root in water for 15-20 minutes to make a decoction. Licorice root decoction can help soothe the stomach lining and reduce inflammation.

Marshmallow Root Infusion: Steep marshmallow root in hot water for marshmallow root infusion. Marshmallow root infusion has demulcent properties, which can help soothe and protect the digestive tract.

- Slippery Elm Bark Powder: Mix slippery elm bark powder with water to form a gel-like substance. Slippery elm bark powder can help soothe irritated digestive tissues and relieve symptoms of heartburn and gastritis.
- Artichoke Leaf Extract: Steep artichoke leaves in hot water for artichoke leaf extract. Artichoke leaf extract can help improve digestion by increasing bile production and reducing symptoms of indigestion.

Coriander Seed Tea: Crush coriander seeds and steep them in hot water for coriander seed tea. Coriander seed tea can help relieve gas, bloating, and indigestion.

Cumin Seed Infusion: Crush cumin seeds and steep them in hot water for cumin seed infusion. Cumin seed infusion can help stimulate digestion and relieve symptoms of indigestion.

Angelica Root Tincture: Prepare a tincture using angelica root and alcohol. Angelica root tincture can help stimulate digestion and relieve symptoms of indigestion.

Caraway Seed Tea: Crush caraway seeds and steep them in hot water for caraway seed tea. Caraway seed tea can help relieve gas, bloating, and indigestion.

Remember to consult with a healthcare professional before using any herbal remedies, especially if you have underlying health conditions or are pregnant or breastfeeding. These DIY herbal digestive remedies can complement a healthy lifestyle but should not replace medical treatment if you have serious digestive issues.

1. Adaptogenic Herbs for Stress Management

Adaptogenic herbs are known for their ability to help the body adapt to stress and maintain balance. Here are some popular adaptogenic herbs for stress management:

- Ashwagandha (Withania somnifera): Ashwagandha is one of the most well-known adaptogenic herbs. It helps the body cope with stress by reducing cortisol levels and promoting relaxation. It's often used to improve energy levels, enhance mental clarity, and support overall well-being.
- Rhodiola (Rhodiola rosea): Rhodiola is another popular adaptogen that helps the body adapt to stress and increase resilience. It's known for its ability to improve energy levels, enhance mental focus, and reduce fatigue. Rhodiola is often used to support cognitive function and promote a sense of calmness.
- Holy Basil (Ocimum sanctum): Also known as Tulsi, holy basil is revered in Ayurvedic medicine for its stress-relieving properties. It helps the body cope with stress by reducing cortisol levels and promoting relaxation. Holy basil is often used to support mental clarity, uplift mood, and promote overall well-being.
- Siberian Ginseng (Eleutherococcus senticosus): Siberian ginseng is an adaptogenic herb that helps the body adapt to stress and increase resilience. It's known for its ability to enhance physical performance, improve stamina, and reduce

fatigue. Siberian ginseng is often used to support immune function and promote overall vitality.

- Schisandra (Schisandra chinensis): Schisandra is an adaptogenic herb that helps the body cope with stress and increase resilience. It's known for its ability to enhance mental clarity, improve focus, and reduce fatigue. Schisandra is often used to support liver function and promote overall well-being.

- Licorice Root (Glycyrrhiza glabra): Licorice root is an adaptogenic herb that helps the body cope with stress and increase resilience. It's known for its ability to support adrenal function, balance cortisol levels, and promote relaxation. Licorice root is often used to support digestive health and promote overall vitality.

- Reishi Mushroom (Ganoderma lucidum): Reishi mushroom is an adaptogenic herb that helps the body cope with stress and increase resilience. It's known for its calming effects, immune-boosting properties, and ability to promote overall well-being. Reishi mushroom is often used to support cardiovascular health and promote longevity.

- Cordyceps (Cordyceps sinensis): Cordyceps is an adaptogenic herb that helps the body cope with stress and increase resilience. It's known for its energy-boosting properties, endurance-enhancing effects, and ability to reduce fatigue. Cordyceps is often used to support athletic performance and promote overall vitality.

These adaptogenic herbs can be consumed in various forms, including teas, tinctures, capsules, and powders. It's important to consult with a healthcare professional before incorporating adaptogenic herbs into your routine, especially if you have any underlying health conditions or are pregnant or breastfeeding.

2. Relaxing Herbal Infusions and Tinctures

Here are some relaxing herbal infusions and tinctures that can help promote relaxation and reduce stress:

- Chamomile Tea: Chamomile is well-known for its calming properties. Steep dried chamomile flowers in hot water for a few minutes to make a soothing tea that can help relax the mind and body.
- Lavender Infusion: Lavender is a fragrant herb that has been used for centuries to promote relaxation. Steep dried lavender flowers in hot water to make a calming infusion. You can also add a few drops of lavender essential oil to a carrier oil for a relaxing massage.
- Valerian Root Tincture: Valerian root is a potent herb that is commonly used to promote relaxation and improve sleep quality. Prepare a valerian root tincture by soaking dried valerian root in alcohol for several weeks. Take a few drops of the tincture before bedtime to help calm the nervous system and induce sleep.
- Passionflower Tea: Passionflower is a gentle herb that can help reduce anxiety and promote relaxation. Steep dried passion flower leaves in hot water for a few minutes to make a soothing tea that can help calm the mind and body.
- Lemon Balm Tincture: Lemon balm is a calming herb that can help reduce stress and anxiety. Prepare a lemon balm tincture by soaking dried lemon balm leaves in alcohol for several weeks. Take a few drops of the tincture as needed to help promote relaxation.

- Skullcap Infusion: Skullcap is a relaxing herb that can help calm the nervous system and promote relaxation. Steep dried skullcap leaves in hot water for a few minutes to make a soothing infusion that can help reduce stress and anxiety.
- Kava Kava Tincture: Kava kava is a powerful herb that is commonly used to promote relaxation and reduce anxiety. Prepare a kava kava tincture by soaking dried kava kava root in alcohol for several weeks. Take a few drops of the tincture as needed to help calm the mind and body.
- Catnip Tea: Catnip is a gentle herb that can help promote relaxation and reduce stress. Steep dried catnip leaves in hot water for a few minutes to make a soothing tea that can help calm the nervous system.
- California Poppy Tincture: California poppy is a mild sedative herb that can help promote relaxation and improve sleep quality. Prepare a California poppy tincture by soaking dried California poppy leaves in alcohol for several weeks. Take a few drops of the tincture before bedtime to help induce sleep.
- Rose Tea: Rose petals have a calming effect on the mind and body. Steep dried rose petals in hot water for a few minutes to make a fragrant tea that can help promote relaxation and reduce stress.

These relaxing herbal infusions and tinctures can be enjoyed throughout the day or before bedtime to help promote relaxation and reduce stress. As always, consult with a healthcare professional before using any herbal remedies, especially if you have any underlying health conditions or are pregnant or breastfeeding.

D. Pain Management

1. Analgesic Herbs for Natural Pain Relief

Here is a list of herbs that are commonly used for pain management:

- Turmeric (Curcuma longa): Turmeric contains a compound called curcumin, which has anti-inflammatory properties. It is often used to alleviate pain associated with conditions such as arthritis and muscle soreness.
- Ginger (Zingiber officinale): Ginger has anti-inflammatory and analgesic properties, making it effective for relieving various types of pain, including muscle pain, arthritis pain, and menstrual cramps.
- White Willow Bark (Salix alba): White willow bark contains salicin, which is similar to aspirin and has pain-relieving properties. It is often used to relieve headaches, back pain, and arthritis pain.
- Devil's Claw (Harpagophytum procumbens): Devil's claw has anti-inflammatory and analgesic properties and is commonly used to relieve pain associated with conditions such as arthritis, back pain, and muscle pain.

- Boswellia (Boswellia serrata): Boswellia contains compounds that have anti-inflammatory properties, making it effective for relieving pain associated with conditions such as arthritis and inflammatory bowel disease.
- Arnica (Arnica montana): Arnica is often used topically to relieve pain and inflammation associated with bruises, sprains, and muscle soreness.

- Capsaicin (Capsicum annuum): Capsaicin is the active component in chili peppers and is often used topically in creams and ointments to relieve pain associated with conditions such as arthritis, neuropathy, and muscle pain.
- Kratom (Mitragyna speciosa): Kratom contains alkaloids that have analgesic properties and is commonly used to relieve chronic pain, including pain associated with conditions such as fibromyalgia and arthritis.

- St. John's Wort (Hypericum perforatum): St. John's Wort has anti-inflammatory and analgesic properties and is often used to relieve nerve pain, muscle pain, and pain associated with conditions such as sciatica and shingles.
- Cloves (Syzygium aromaticum): Cloves contain eugenol, which has analgesic properties and is often used to relieve toothaches and gum pain. Clove oil can be applied topically or used in mouth rinses.
- Chamomile (Matricaria chamomilla): Chamomile has anti-inflammatory and analgesic properties and is often used to relieve muscle spasms, menstrual cramps, and tension headaches.

These herbs can be used individually or in combination to manage various types of pain. However, it's important to consult with a healthcare professional before using any herbal remedies, especially if you have any underlying health conditions or are pregnant or breastfeeding.

2. Herbal Compresses and Salves

- **Arnica Salve:** Arnica salve is made by infusing arnica flowers in oil and combining it with beeswax to create a soothing balm. It's commonly used to relieve muscle pain, bruising, and inflammation.

- **Comfrey Salve:** Comfrey is known for its wound-healing properties and is often used in salves to promote tissue repair and reduce inflammation. Comfrey salve can be used to alleviate pain and promote healing of bruises, sprains, and minor wounds.
- **Cayenne Salve:** Cayenne contains capsaicin, which has analgesic properties and can help relieve muscle and joint pain. Cayenne salve is commonly used to alleviate arthritis pain, muscle soreness, and neuropathy.
- **Plantain Salve:** Plantain has anti-inflammatory and wound-healing properties and is often used in salves to soothe skin irritations, insect bites, and minor cuts. Plantain salve can help reduce pain and promote healing of damaged skin.

- **St. John's Wort Salve:** St. John's Wort has anti-inflammatory and analgesic properties and is commonly used in salves to relieve nerve pain, muscle pain, and inflammation. St. John's Wort salve can be used topically to alleviate pain and promote healing.

These herbal compresses and salves can be made at home using dried or fresh herbs, carrier oils, and beeswax. However, it's important to research and follow proper procedures when making herbal remedies to ensure safety and effectiveness. Additionally, consult with a healthcare professional before using any herbal remedies, especially if you have any underlying health conditions or are pregnant or breastfeeding.

- **Eucalyptus (Eucalyptus globulus):** Eucalyptus leaves contain cineole, which has mucolytic and expectorant properties, making it useful for respiratory conditions such as coughs, colds, and congestion. Eucalyptus oil can be used in steam inhalation or diluted in carrier oil for chest rubs.
- **Peppermint (Mentha × piperita):** Peppermint contains menthol, which acts as a decongestant and helps to soothe

respiratory passages. Peppermint tea, inhalation of peppermint oil, or throat lozenges can help alleviate symptoms of respiratory congestion and irritation.

- **Thyme (Thymus vulgaris):** Thyme contains thymol, which has antiseptic and expectorant properties. Thyme tea or steam inhalation with thyme oil can help relieve coughs, bronchitis, and congestion.

- **Ginger (Zingiber officinale):** Ginger has anti-inflammatory and antimicrobial properties, which can help soothe sore throats and reduce coughing. Ginger tea or adding ginger to meals can provide respiratory support.

- **Licorice Root (Glycyrrhiza glabra):** Licorice root has demulcent and expectorant properties, making it useful for soothing irritated throats and reducing coughing. Licorice root tea or lozenges can help alleviate respiratory symptoms.

- **Oregano (Origanum vulgare):** Oregano contains carvacrol and rosmarinic acid, which have antimicrobial and anti-inflammatory properties. Oregano tea or steam inhalation with oregano oil can help fight respiratory infections and reduce inflammation.

- **Marshmallow Root (Althaea officinalis):** Marshmallow root has demulcent properties, which can help soothe irritated throats and reduce coughing. Marshmallow root tea or lozenges can provide relief for respiratory conditions.

- **Garlic (Allium sativum):** Garlic contains allicin, which has antimicrobial properties. Consuming garlic can help boost the immune system and fight respiratory infections.

- **Lemon (Citrus limon):** Lemon contains vitamin C, which can help support the immune system and reduce the severity of respiratory infections. Drinking lemon water or adding lemon to tea can provide respiratory support.

- **Chamomile (Matricaria chamomilla)**: Chamomile has anti-inflammatory properties and can help soothe irritated throats and reduce coughing. Chamomile tea or steam inhalation with chamomile oil can provide respiratory relief.

These herbs can be used individually or in combination to support respiratory health and alleviate symptoms of respiratory conditions. However, it's important to consult with a healthcare professional before using any herbal remedies, especially if you have any underlying health conditions or are pregnant or breastfeeding.

2. Herbal Steam Inhalations and Syrups

- **Eucalyptus:** Add a few drops of eucalyptus essential oil to a bowl of hot water. Lean over the bowl with a towel covering your head to inhale the steam. Eucalyptus steam inhalation helps clear congestion and relieve respiratory symptoms.
- **Peppermint:** Steep fresh or dried peppermint leaves in hot water, then pour the infusion into a bowl. Lean over the bowl and cover your head with a towel to inhale the peppermint steam. Peppermint steam inhalation can help soothe respiratory irritation and clear nasal passages.
- **Thyme:** Steep fresh or dried thyme leaves in hot water, then strain the infusion into a bowl. Inhale the thyme steam by covering your head with a towel and leaning over the bowl. Thyme steam inhalation is beneficial for relieving coughs, congestion, and respiratory infections.

- **Rosemary:** Boil fresh or dried rosemary in water, then transfer the mixture to a bowl. Inhale the rosemary steam by covering your head with a towel and leaning over the bowl. Rosemary steam inhalation can help open up airways and relieve respiratory congestion.

- **Lavender:** Add a few drops of lavender essential oil to hot water in a bowl. Inhale the lavender steam by covering your head with a towel and leaning over the bowl. Lavender steam inhalation can promote relaxation and relieve respiratory symptoms.

Herbal Syrups:

- **Honey and Lemon:** Mix equal parts of honey and freshly squeezed lemon juice to create a soothing syrup. Honey and lemon syrup can help soothe sore throats, suppress coughs, and provide immune support.
- **Ginger and Honey:** Steep fresh ginger slices in hot water to make a ginger infusion, then mix it with honey to create a syrup. Ginger and honey syrup can help relieve coughs, sore throats, and respiratory congestion.
- **Elderberry:** Cook elderberries with water and honey to make an elderberry syrup. Elderberry syrup is rich in antioxidants and can help boost the immune system, reduce inflammation, and relieve respiratory symptoms.
- **Marshmallow Root:** Steep marshmallow root in hot water to make a decoction, then mix it with honey to create a soothing syrup. Marshmallow root syrup can help soothe sore throats, relieve coughs, and reduce respiratory irritation.
- **Licorice Root:** Steep licorice root in hot water to make a decoction, then mix it with honey to create a sweet syrup. Licorice root syrup can help soothe sore throats, suppress coughs, and reduce respiratory inflammation.

These herbal steam inhalations and syrups can provide natural relief for respiratory symptoms and promote overall respiratory health. However, it's important to consult with a healthcare professional before using any herbal remedies, especially if you have any underlying health conditions or are pregnant or breastfeeding.

D. Men's Health

Saw Palmetto (Serenoa repens):

- Commonly used to support prostate health and alleviate symptoms of benign prostatic hyperplasia (BPH).
- Helps reduce urinary frequency, urgency, and nighttime urination.
- Supports hormonal balance and may inhibit the conversion of testosterone to dihydrotestosterone (DHT).

Pygeum (Prunus africana):

- Supports prostate health and may reduce symptoms of BPH, such as urinary frequency and incomplete emptying of the bladder.
- Has anti-inflammatory properties that help reduce prostate swelling and improve urinary flow.

Nettle Root (Urtica dioica):

- Contains compounds that help reduce inflammation and support prostate health.
- May help alleviate symptoms of BPH, including urinary retention and decreased urinary flow.
- Supports hormonal balance and may inhibit the enzyme responsible for converting testosterone to DHT.

Pumpkin Seed (Cucurbita pepo):

- Rich in zinc, which is essential for prostate health and hormone regulation.
- Contains phytosterols that help reduce inflammation and support urinary function.
- May help alleviate symptoms of BPH, such as urinary urgency and frequency.

Stinging Nettle (Urtica dioica):

- Has diuretic properties that help reduce urinary symptoms associated with BPH.
- Contains compounds that help reduce inflammation and support prostate health.
- May help improve urinary flow and reduce nighttime urination.

Green Tea (Camellia sinensis):

- Rich in antioxidants called catechins, which help reduce inflammation and support prostate health.
- May help inhibit the growth of prostate cancer cells and reduce the risk of developing prostate cancer.
- Supports overall immune function and may reduce the risk of prostate infections.

Turmeric (Curcuma longa):

- Contains curcumin, which has anti-inflammatory and antioxidant properties.
- May help reduce inflammation in the prostate gland and alleviate symptoms of BPH.
- Supports overall prostate health and may reduce the risk of prostate cancer.

Ginger (Zingiber officinale):

- Has anti-inflammatory properties that help reduce prostate inflammation and alleviate symptoms of BPH.
- Supports overall urinary function and may reduce urinary symptoms associated with prostate enlargement.
- Supports immune function and may reduce the risk of prostate infections.

Garlic (Allium sativum):

- Contains compounds that help reduce inflammation and support prostate health.
- Supports overall immune function and may reduce the risk of prostate infections.
- May help reduce the risk of developing prostate cancer.

Red Clover (Trifolium pratense):

- Contains isoflavones that help balance hormone levels and support prostate health.
- May help reduce symptoms of BPH, such as urinary urgency and frequency.
- Supports overall immune function and may reduce the risk of prostate infections.

These herbs can be consumed as teas, tinctures, or supplements to support prostate health and vitality. However, it's important to consult with a healthcare professional before using any herbal remedies, especially if you have any underlying health conditions or are taking medications

2. Herbal Tonics for Male Wellness

Tribulus Terrestris Tonic:

- Supports testosterone production and libido.
- Helps improve muscle strength and endurance.
- May enhance overall vitality and energy levels.

Maca Root Tonic:

- Supports hormone balance and libido.
- Helps increase stamina and endurance.
- May improve fertility and reproductive health.

Ashwagandha Tonic:

- Adaptogenic herb that helps reduce stress and anxiety.
- Supports hormone balance and libido.
- Enhances energy levels and overall vitality.

Ginseng Tonic:

- Adaptogenic herb that helps increase energy and stamina.
- Supports hormone balance and libido.
- May improve cognitive function and mental clarity.

Horny Goat Weed Tonic:

- Supports libido and sexual function.
- Helps improve blood flow and erectile function.
- May enhance overall energy and vitality.

Saw Palmetto Tonic:

- Supports prostate health and hormone balance.
- Helps alleviate symptoms of benign prostatic hyperplasia (BPH).
- May support urinary function and overall male wellness.

Nettle Root Tonic:

- Supports prostate health and hormone balance.
- Helps reduce inflammation and support urinary function.
- May enhance overall vitality and energy levels.

Tongkat Ali Tonic:

- Supports testosterone production and libido.
- Helps improve muscle mass and strength.
- May enhance overall male wellness and vitality.

Ginkgo Biloba Tonic:

- Supports cognitive function and mental clarity.
- Improves blood flow and circulation.
- May enhance sexual function and overall male wellness.

Damiana Leaf Tonic:

- Supports libido and sexual function.
- Helps reduce stress and anxiety.
- May enhance overall energy and vitality.

These herbal tonics can be consumed as teas, tinctures, or supplements to support male wellness. However, it's important to consult with a healthcare professional before using any herbal remedies, especially if you have any underlying health conditions or are taking medications.

V. Herbal Remedies for Children and Families

Chamomile Tea:

- Helps calm and soothe children, promoting relaxation and better sleep.
- Relieves symptoms of colic, gas, and upset stomach.
- Safe for children when used in appropriate doses.

Peppermint Oil:

- Relieves nausea and indigestion in children.
- Can be diluted and applied topically to soothe headaches and muscle aches.
- Not recommended for children under six years old.

Honey and Lemon:

- Soothes sore throats and coughs in children.
- Honey has antimicrobial properties, while lemon provides vitamin C.
- Not recommended for children under one year old due to the risk of botulism.

Ginger Chews or Tea:

- Relieves nausea and motion sickness in children.
- Helps ease stomach discomfort and improve digestion.
- Suitable for children over two years old.

Echinacea Tincture or Tea:

- Boosts the immune system and helps fight off colds and flu.
- Can shorten the duration and severity of illness in children.
- Not recommended for prolonged use or children with autoimmune disorders.

Arnica Cream or Gel:

- Relieves pain and inflammation from bruises, sprains, and muscle strains.
- Safe for topical use in children, but avoid open wounds or broken skin.
- Not for internal use or ingestion.

Calendula Cream:

- Soothes and heals minor cuts, scrapes, and insect bites in children.
- Promotes skin healing and reduces inflammation.
- Safe for topical use in children of all ages.

Lavender Oil:

- Promotes relaxation and improves sleep quality in children.
- Helps soothe skin irritations and minor burns.
- Dilute before topical application and avoid contact with eyes.

Eucalyptus Oil:

- Relieves congestion and improves breathing during colds and respiratory infections.
- Dilute and use in a diffuser or steam inhalation for children over six years old.
- Avoid direct contact with the skin and mucous membranes.

Fennel Tea:

- Relieves colic, gas, and digestive discomfort in infants and young children.
- Soothes stomach cramps and promotes healthy digestion.
- Use cautiously and in small amounts for infants and young children.

These herbal remedies can be used safely for children and families when used appropriately and in moderation. However, it's important to consult with a pediatrician or healthcare professional before introducing any new herbal remedies, especially if your child has underlying health conditions or is taking medications.

A.Safe Herbs for Children

Chamomile (Matricaria chamomilla):

- Soothes upset stomach, colic, and teething discomfort.
- Helps promote relaxation and better sleep.
- Safe for children when used in appropriate doses.

Peppermint (Mentha piperita):

- Relieves symptoms of indigestion, gas, and bloating.
- Can ease nausea and improve digestion.
- Safe for children over two years old in diluted forms.

Ginger (Zingiber officinale):

- Helps relieve nausea, motion sickness, and upset stomach.
- Can be used to improve digestion and reduce gas.
- Safe for children over two years old in small doses.

Lemon Balm (Melissa officinalis):

- Calms nerves and reduces anxiety in children.
- Helps promote relaxation and improve sleep quality.
- Safe for children when used in moderation.

Lavender (Lavandula angustifolia):

- Promotes relaxation and helps improve sleep.
- Soothes skin irritations and minor burns.
- Safe for children when used topically or inhaled.

Echinacea (Echinacea purpurea):

- Boosts the immune system and helps fight off colds and flu.
- Shortens the duration and severity of illness in children.
- Safe for short-term use in children over two years old.

Calendula (Calendula officinalis):

- Soothes and heals minor cuts, scrapes, and insect bites.
- Promotes skin healing and reduces inflammation.
- Safe for topical use in children of all ages.

Marshmallow (Althaea officinalis):

- Relieves sore throat and dry cough in children.
- Soothes mucous membranes and promotes healing.
- Safe for children when used in appropriate forms.

Nettle (Urtica dioica):

- Supports overall health and provides essential nutrients.

- Relieves seasonal allergies and hay fever symptoms.
- Safe for children when prepared as a tea or consumed in food.

Fennel (Foeniculum vulgare):

- Relieves colic, gas, and digestive discomfort in infants.
- Soothes stomach cramps and promotes healthy digestion.
- Safe for infants and young children in small amounts.

These herbs can be used safely for children when used appropriately and in moderation. However, it's important to consult with a pediatrician or healthcare professional before introducing any new herbal remedies, especially if your child has underlying health conditions or is taking medications.

B. Integrating Herbal Medicine into Family Life

Educate Yourself About Herbs:

- Research different herbs and their uses.
- Learn about safety precautions and proper dosage for each herb.
- Consider taking herbal medicine courses or workshops.

Start with Simple Remedies:

- Begin with commonly used and well-understood herbs.
- Focus on herbs that address minor ailments like colds, digestive issues, or skin irritations.
- Gradually expand your herbal repertoire as you gain more experience and confidence.

Create a Family Herbal Medicine Kit:

- Gather essential herbal remedies for common ailments.
- Include items such as chamomile tea, peppermint oil, arnica salve, and elderberry syrup.
- Store herbs and herbal products in a designated area, keeping them out of reach of children.

Teach Children About Herbs:

- Involve children in herbal preparations and remedies.
- Teach them about the properties and uses of different herbs.
- Encourage them to participate in gardening or foraging for herbs.

Practice Prevention:

- Use herbs to support overall health and wellness.
- Incorporate immune-boosting herbs into your family's diet, such as garlic, ginger, and echinacea.
- Explore herbal teas and tonics to promote relaxation and stress relief.

Integrate Herbs into Daily Life:

- Use herbs in cooking and meal preparation.
- Incorporate herbal teas into your family's beverage choices.
- Create herbal-infused oils, salves, or balms for skincare and minor first aid needs.

Consult with a Professional:

- Seek guidance from a qualified herbalist or naturopathic doctor.
- Consult healthcare professionals, especially when dealing with serious health issues or if you're unsure about using herbs for specific conditions.

- Keep your primary care provider informed about any herbal remedies your family is using.

Practice Safety and Caution:

- Research potential interactions between herbs and medications.
- Start with small doses when trying new herbs, especially for children.
- Monitor for any adverse reactions and discontinue use if necessary.

Keep Records and Notes:

- Maintain a journal or notebook to track your family's experiences with herbal remedies.
- Note which herbs work well for specific ailments and any dosages used.
- Document any adverse reactions or unexpected outcomes for future reference.

Embrace Holistic Wellness:

- Integrate herbal medicine with other holistic health practices, such as healthy nutrition, regular exercise, and mindfulness.
- Encourage open communication and shared decision-making within your family regarding health and wellness choices.

By integrating herbal medicine into family life in a thoughtful and informed manner, you can empower your family to take a proactive approach to health and well-being while fostering a deeper connection to nature and traditional healing practices.

VI. Growing and Harvesting Medicinal Herbs

A. Creating a Herbal Garden

I. Planning Your Herbal Garden

- Choose a suitable location with ample sunlight and well-drained soil.
- Determine the size and layout of your garden based on available space and herb varieties.
- Research herbs that thrive in your climate and consider their growth habits and space requirements.
- Design the garden layout, keeping in mind factors like companion planting and accessibility.

II. Preparing the Soil

- Test the soil pH and nutrient levels to assess its fertility and suitability for growing herbs.
- Amend the soil with organic matter such as compost, aged manure, or peat moss to improve soil structure and fertility.
- Use a garden fork or tiller to loosen the soil and remove any weeds or debris.

III. Planting Your Herbal Garden

- Start seeds indoors several weeks before the last frost date in your area, following specific planting instructions for each herb.

- Directly sow seeds into the garden according to recommended spacing and depth, ensuring adequate room for growth.
- Transplant seedlings into the garden, gently loosening roots and watering thoroughly to promote establishment.

IV. Caring for Your Herbal Garden

- Provide consistent watering, keeping the soil evenly moist but not waterlogged.
- Apply mulch around plants to retain moisture, suppress weeds, and regulate soil temperature.
- Fertilize herbs with organic fertilizers or compost to provide essential nutrients for healthy growth.
- Prune herbs regularly to encourage bushy growth and remove any dead or damaged foliage.

V. Managing Pests and Diseases

- Monitor the garden for signs of pests such as aphids, slugs, or caterpillars, and take appropriate action to control infestations.
- Use natural pest control methods such as companion planting, beneficial insects, or organic pesticides.
- Practice good garden hygiene by removing diseased plants, rotating crops, and maintaining proper spacing to prevent the spread of diseases.

VI. Harvesting Your Herbal Garden

- Time your harvest for optimal flavor and potency, typically in the morning after dew has dried but before the heat of the day.
- Use sharp scissors or pruning shears to make clean cuts, harvesting leaves, flowers, or seeds as needed.

- Dry herbs for long-term storage by hanging them in bundles, using a dehydrator, or air-drying them on screens.
- Store dried herbs in airtight containers in a cool, dark place to maintain their flavor and potency.

VII. Continual Care and Maintenance

- Regularly weed the garden, monitor for pests and diseases, and provide ongoing care as needed to ensure the health of your herbs.
- Rotate herb crops annually to prevent soil depletion and reduce the risk of pest and disease buildup.
- Stay curious and open to trying new herbs and cultivation techniques, and keep a gardening journal to track your progress.

VIII. Enjoying the Fruits of Your Labor

- Incorporate fresh herbs into your cooking to enhance flavor and nutrition.
- Use herbs for homemade teas, tinctures, salves, and other natural remedies to support health and wellness.
- Share your herbal bounty with friends, family, and neighbors, and spread the joy of gardening and herbalism.

By following these steps, you can create and maintain a thriving herbal garden that provides beauty, flavor, and health benefits for you and your family.

B. Harvesting and Drying Herbs

1. **Choose the Right Time to Harvest**:

- Harvest herbs in the morning after dew has evaporated but before the heat of the day.

- Choose a day when the weather is dry to minimize moisture content in the herbs.

2. **Prepare Your Tools**:

- Gather sharp scissors, pruning shears, or a small knife for harvesting.

- Bring a clean basket or tray to collect the harvested herbs.

3. **Harvesting the Herbs**:

1. Identify the parts of the herb to harvest (leaves, flowers, seeds, etc.).

2. Cut or pinch off the herb stems just above a set of healthy leaves or buds.

3. Avoid harvesting more than one-third of the plant's growth to ensure its continued health and vitality.

4. Remove any damaged, discolored, or diseased parts of the plant while harvesting.

4. **Handling and Cleaning**:

- Handle the harvested herbs gently to avoid bruising or damaging them.

- Shake off any excess dirt or debris from the herbs.

- Rinse the herbs lightly with cool water if necessary, but avoid soaking them, as excess moisture can lead to mold during drying.

5. **Drying Methods**:

1. Air Drying:

   - Bundle small bunches of herbs together and secure them with twine or rubber bands.

   - Hang the bundles upside down in a warm, dry, well-ventilated area out of direct sunlight.

   - Alternatively, spread the herbs in a single layer on a clean screen or drying rack.

2. Oven Drying:

   - Place herbs on a baking sheet lined with parchment paper, making sure they are in a single layer.

   - Set the oven to its lowest temperature (usually around 100-120°F or 40-50°C) and prop the oven door open slightly.

   - Check the herbs frequently to prevent them from overheating or burning.

3. Dehydrator:

- Arrange herbs in a single layer on dehydrator trays, leaving space between each piece for air circulation.

- Set the dehydrator to the appropriate temperature for drying herbs (usually between 95-110°F or 35-45°C).

- Check the herbs periodically until they are thoroughly dry.

6. **Monitoring and Testing**:

- Check the herbs regularly during the drying process for signs of mold or moisture.

- To test for dryness, try crushing a small amount of the herb between your fingers. It should crumble easily when fully dry.

7. **Storing Dried Herbs**:

- Once the herbs are completely dry, remove the leaves or flowers from the stems if desired.

- Store the dried herbs in airtight containers such as glass jars or resealable bags.

- Label the containers with the name of the herb and the date of harvesting to keep track of freshness.

8. **Using Dried Herbs**:

- Use dried herbs in cooking, teas, herbal remedies, and crafts as desired.

- Store dried herbs in a cool, dark place away from heat and sunlight to maintain their flavor and potency.

By following these steps, you can effectively harvest and dry herbs to preserve their flavor and medicinal properties for future use.

C. Preserving Herbs for Long-Term Use

1. **Choosing Herbs for Preservation**:

   - Select fresh, healthy herbs from your garden or local market.

   - Harvest herbs at their peak flavor and potency for the best results.

   - Consider the intended use of the herbs when choosing which ones to preserve.

2. **Methods of Preservation**:

   1. Drying:

   - Air drying: Hang bundles of herbs upside down in a warm, well-ventilated area until completely dry.

   - Oven drying: Arrange herbs on a baking sheet and dry them in a low-temperature oven with the door slightly ajar.

   - Dehydrating: Use a food dehydrator to dry herbs quickly and efficiently at a low temperature.

   2. Freezing:

- Freeze whole or chopped herbs in ice cube trays filled with water or olive oil.

- Alternatively, spread herbs in a single layer on a baking sheet and freeze them before transferring to freezer bags or containers.

3. Infusing:

- Make herbal infusions by steeping fresh or dried herbs in oil, vinegar, or alcohol to extract their flavors and medicinal properties.

- Store infused oils and vinegars in tightly sealed bottles or jars in a cool, dark place.

4. Salting:

- Layer fresh herbs with coarse salt in a clean, dry jar, alternating between layers until the jar is full.

- Store the jar in a cool, dark place and use the preserved herbs as a seasoning or flavor enhancer.

3. **Preparing Herbs for Preservation**:

- Wash fresh herbs gently in cold water and pat them dry with paper towels to remove any dirt or debris.

- Remove any damaged or discolored leaves and trim the stems as needed.

- For drying, bundle herbs together and tie them with twine or rubber bands before hanging or laying them out for drying.

4. **Storing Preserved Herbs**:

   - Label containers with the name of the herb and the date of preservation to keep track of freshness.

   - Store dried herbs in airtight containers such as glass jars or resealable bags in a cool, dark place away from heat and moisture.

   - Freeze herbs in portion-sized containers or bags for easy use in cooking and recipes.

   - Keep infused oils and vinegars tightly sealed and store them in a cool, dark place to prevent spoilage.

5. **Using Preserved Herbs**:

   - Use dried herbs in cooking, teas, herbal remedies, and crafts as desired.

   - Add frozen herbs directly to dishes while cooking or thaw them before use.

   - Incorporate infused oils and vinegars into salad dressings, marinades, sauces, and dips for added flavor.

6. **Monitoring and Refreshing**:

- Periodically check preserved herbs for signs of spoilage, such as mold or off odors.

- Discard any herbs that show signs of spoilage and refresh your supply as needed by preserving fresh batches.

By following these steps, you can effectively preserve herbs for long-term use, ensuring that you have a steady supply of flavorful and aromatic herbs year-round.

VII. Advanced Herbal Medicine Techniques

A. Herbal Extracts and Tinctures

1. **Gather Your Materials**:

   - Dried herbs or fresh herbs that have been thoroughly cleaned and dried.

   - High-proof alcohol such as vodka, brandy, or grain alcohol (at least 80 proof).

   - Glass jars with tight-fitting lids for macerating the herbs.

   - Glass dropper bottles for storing the finished tinctures.

   - Labels and markers to identify the herbs and date of preparation.

2. **Selecting Herbs**:

- Choose high-quality herbs that are suitable for making extracts or tinctures.

- Consider the medicinal properties and intended use of the herbs when selecting which ones to use.

- Ensure that the herbs are thoroughly dried to prevent spoilage and mold growth.

3. **Preparing the Herbs**:

- If using fresh herbs, chop them into small pieces to increase surface area for extraction.

- If using dried herbs, crush or grind them to release their aromatic oils and active compounds.

- Fill a glass jar with the prepared herbs, leaving some space at the top for the alcohol.

4. **Creating the Extract or Tincture**:

- Pour the alcohol over the herbs in the jar, making sure they are completely submerged.

- Use a clean spoon or chopstick to press down on the herbs and release any air bubbles.

- Seal the jar tightly with a lid and shake it gently to mix the alcohol and herbs.

5. **Macerating the Mixture**:

   - Place the jar in a cool, dark place away from direct sunlight.

   - Allow the herbs to macerate in the alcohol for at least 4-6 weeks, shaking the jar gently every few days to agitate the mixture.

   - The longer the herbs macerate, the stronger the tincture will be.

6. **Straining the Tincture**:

   - After the maceration period is complete, strain the tincture through a fine mesh strainer or cheesecloth into a clean glass container.

   - Squeeze out as much liquid as possible from the herbs to extract all of their medicinal properties.

7. **Bottling and Storage**:

   - Transfer the strained tincture into glass dropper bottles for easy dispensing.

   - Label the bottles with the name of the herb, date of preparation, and any other relevant information.

   - Store the tinctures in a cool, dark place away from heat and sunlight to preserve their potency.

8. **Using the Tinctures**:

- Take tinctures orally by diluting them in water or juice before consumption.

- Follow recommended dosage guidelines for each herb and consult with a healthcare professional if unsure.

- Tinctures can also be added to teas, herbal preparations, or used topically for certain conditions.

9. **Experimenting and Adjusting**:

- Feel free to experiment with different herbs and alcohol ratios to create custom tinctures tailored to your specific needs.

- Keep notes on the strength and effectiveness of each tincture for future reference and adjustments.

10. **Safety Considerations**:

- Be aware of any potential interactions between herbs and medications, and consult with a healthcare professional before using herbal tinctures, especially if pregnant, breastfeeding, or have any underlying health conditions.

- Always use clean, sterilized equipment and jars to prevent contamination and spoilage of the tinctures.

By following these steps, you can create high-quality herbal extracts and tinctures that preserve the medicinal properties of the herbs for long-term use.

B. Herbal Poultices and Compresses

1. **Gather Your Materials**:

   - Fresh or dried herbs of your choice (such as chamomile, calendula, comfrey, or plantain).

   - Clean cloth or gauze pads for making the poultice or compress.

   - Hot water for soaking the herbs (if using dried herbs).

   - Mortar and pestle or blender for grinding fresh herbs (if using fresh herbs).

   - Optional: Essential oils or carrier oils for added therapeutic benefits.

2. **Selecting Herbs**:

   - Choose herbs with properties that match the intended use of the poultice or compress (e.g., anti-inflammatory, analgesic, or wound-healing).

   - Consider using a single herb or combining multiple herbs for synergistic effects.

3. **Preparing the Herbs**:

   - If using dried herbs, place them in a bowl and cover them with hot water. Let them soak for a few minutes until they become soft and pliable.

- If using fresh herbs, grind or crush them using a mortar and pestle or blender to release their juices and active compounds.

4. **Creating the Poultice**:

1. For fresh herbs:

   - Place the crushed or ground herbs directly onto a clean cloth or gauze pad.

   - Spread the herbs evenly over the cloth, leaving space around the edges to fold it over.

2. For dried herbs:

   - Place the softened herbs onto a clean cloth or gauze pad, spreading them evenly.

   - If desired, add a few drops of water to the herbs to create a paste-like consistency.

5. **Applying the Poultice**:

 - Place the poultice directly onto the affected area of the skin.

 - Ensure that the poultice covers the entire area of concern, with a thickness of about ¼ to ½ inch.

 - Secure the poultice in place with a bandage or wrap to keep it from shifting.

6. **Leaving the Poultice On**:

   - Leave the poultice on for 15-30 minutes, or as directed by your healthcare provider.

   - You may experience a warming or tingling sensation as the herbs work to penetrate the skin and provide relief.

7. **Removing and Disposing of the Poultice**:

   - Carefully remove the poultice, taking care not to disturb the affected area.

   - Discard the used herbs and cloth in the compost or trash, as they may contain toxins or contaminants.

8. **Creating a Herbal Compress**:

   1. Steep dried herbs in hot water to create a strong herbal infusion.

   2. Soak a clean cloth or gauze pad in the herbal infusion until fully saturated.

   3. Wring out excess liquid from the cloth and apply it to the affected area.

   4. Leave the compress on for 15-30 minutes, re-soaking it in the herbal infusion as needed to maintain warmth and moisture.

9. **Safety Considerations**:

- Be cautious when using hot poultices or compresses to avoid burns or scalding.

- Discontinue use if you experience any adverse reactions such as redness, itching, or irritation.

- Consult with a healthcare professional before using herbal poultices or compresses, especially if pregnant, breastfeeding, or have any underlying health conditions.

By following these steps, you can effectively create herbal poultices and compresses to provide natural relief for a variety of ailments and promote healing and wellness.

C. Formulating Custom Herbal Remedies

1. **Identify the Purpose of Your Herbal Remedy**:

- Determine the specific health concern or condition you wish to address with the herbal remedy.

- Research the properties and actions of herbs that are known to be effective for your intended purpose.

2. **Choose Suitable Herbs**:

1. Research herbs that are traditionally used for the intended purpose of your remedy.

2. Consider the energetics, taste, and actions of each herb to ensure they complement each other and align with your goals.

3. Select herbs that are readily available, safe for use, and appropriate for the individual's constitution and any existing health conditions.

3. **Plan Your Herbal Formula**:

1. Determine the proportions of each herb in your formula based on their desired effects and potency.

2. Consider whether you will use dried herbs, fresh herbs, or herbal extracts in your formulation.

3. Calculate the total quantity of herbs needed based on the desired batch size of your remedy.

4. **Prepare Your Ingredients**:

- Gather all the herbs and other ingredients needed for your formula.

- If using dried herbs, measure out the appropriate quantities using a scale or measuring spoons.

- If using fresh herbs, wash them thoroughly and chop or grind them as needed.

5. **Combine the Herbs**:

1. Place the measured herbs in a clean glass jar or container.

2. Mix the herbs together thoroughly, ensuring they are evenly distributed throughout the mixture.

3. Consider adding other ingredients such as carrier oils, alcohol, honey, or glycerin to enhance the effectiveness and palatability of your remedy.

6. **Infuse or Extract the Herbs**:

- Choose an appropriate method for extracting the medicinal properties of the herbs, such as making an herbal tea, tincture, oil infusion, or syrup.

- Follow specific instructions for each extraction method, including steeping times, temperatures, and ratios of herbs to solvent.

7. **Strain and Filter**:

- Once the herbs have been infused or extracted, strain the liquid through a fine mesh strainer or cheesecloth to remove any plant material.

- Use a press or squeeze method to extract as much liquid from the herbs as possible.

8. **Bottle and Label Your Remedy**:

- Transfer the strained liquid into clean glass bottles or containers for storage.

- Label each bottle with the name of the remedy, date of preparation, ingredients used, and any relevant dosage or usage instructions.

9. **Store Your Remedy Properly**:

- Store your herbal remedy in a cool, dark place away from heat, light, and moisture to preserve its potency and effectiveness.

- Follow any specific storage recommendations for the type of remedy you have formulated, such as refrigeration for perishable preparations.

10. **Monitor and Adjust**:

- Keep track of the effectiveness of your custom herbal remedy and any feedback from users.

- Adjust the formula as needed based on observed results, changing health conditions, or individual responses.

11. **Seek Professional Guidance**:

- Consult with a qualified herbalist or healthcare provider for personalized guidance and recommendations, especially if formulating remedies for complex health issues or chronic conditions.

By following these steps, you can effectively formulate custom herbal remedies tailored to your specific needs and preferences, promoting health and well-being naturally.

VIII. Herbal Medicine for Mental and Emotional Well-being

A. Herbs for Cognitive Function and Memory

1. **Ginkgo Biloba (Ginkgoaceae)**:

- Improves blood circulation to the brain.

- Enhances memory, concentration, and cognitive function.

- Contains antioxidants that protect brain cells from damage.

- Available in supplement form, typically standardized to contain specific amounts of active compounds.

2. **Bacopa Monnieri (Brahmi)**:

  - Supports memory retention and learning ability.

  - Helps reduce anxiety and stress, which can impair cognitive function.

  - Enhances neurotransmitter function in the brain.

  - Often consumed as a tea or taken in supplement form.

3. **Rosemary (Rosmarinus officinalis)**:

  - Contains compounds that may improve memory and concentration.

  - Acts as a mild stimulant, increasing alertness and mental clarity.

  - Can be used in cooking, aromatherapy, or as a tea.

4. **Turmeric (Curcuma longa)**:

   - Contains curcumin, which has anti-inflammatory and antioxidant
properties.

   - May help improve memory and reduce cognitive decline associated
with aging.

   - Often used in cooking or taken as a supplement.

5. **Sage (Salvia officinalis)**:

   - Improves cognitive function and memory retention.

   - Contains compounds that protect against oxidative stress and
inflammation in the brain.

   - Can be consumed as a tea, added to cooking, or taken as a
supplement.

6. **Gotu Kola (Centella asiatica)**:

   - Enhances cognitive function and memory.

   - Supports overall brain health and circulation.

   - Often used in traditional medicine practices and available in
supplement form.

7. **Lion's Mane Mushroom (Hericium erinaceus)**:

   - Promotes nerve growth factor (NGF) production, which supports
brain health and cognitive function.

   - May help improve memory and focus.

   - Available in supplement form or as a culinary ingredient.

8. **Ashwagandha (Withania somnifera)**:

   - Reduces stress and anxiety, which can impair cognitive function.

   - Supports overall brain health and function.

   - Available in supplement form or as a powder for use in cooking or beverages.

9. **Rhodiola Rosea (Arctic Root or Golden Root)**:

   - Improves mental performance and reduces fatigue.

   - Helps the body adapt to stress and enhances cognitive function.

   - Typically taken in supplement form.

10. **Green Tea (Camellia sinensis)**:

   - Contains caffeine and L-theanine, which can improve alertness, focus, and cognitive function.

   - Rich in antioxidants that protect brain cells from damage.

   - Consumed as a beverage or taken in supplement form.

These herbs can be used individually or in combination to support cognitive function, memory, and overall brain health. It's important to consult with a healthcare professional before adding herbal supplements to your routine, especially if you have any underlying health conditions or are taking medications.

B. Mood-Enhancing Herbs and Herbal Blends

Certainly! Here's a comprehensive guide on mood-enhancing herbs and herbal blends, presented with bullets and numbers:

1. **St. John's Wort (Hypericum perforatum)**:

   - Acts as a natural antidepressant by increasing levels of serotonin, dopamine, and norepinephrine in the brain.

   - Helps alleviate symptoms of mild to moderate depression and mood disorders.

   - Can be taken as a tea, tincture, or standardized extract.

2. **Lavender (Lavandula angustifolia)**:

   - Calms the nervous system and reduces anxiety and stress.

   - Promotes relaxation and improves mood.

   - Often used in aromatherapy, herbal teas, and bath products.

3. **Chamomile (Matricaria chamomilla)**:

- Has mild sedative effects that help reduce anxiety and promote relaxation.

- Improves mood and supports better sleep quality.

- Consumed as a tea, tincture, or added to bathwater.

4. **Lemon Balm (Melissa officinalis)**:

- Relieves stress and anxiety, promoting a sense of calmness and well-being.

- Improves mood and cognitive function.

- Consumed as a tea, tincture, or added to culinary dishes.

5. **Passionflower (Passiflora incarnata)**:

- Acts as a natural sedative and anxiolytic, reducing symptoms of anxiety and depression.

- Promotes relaxation and better sleep quality.

- Available in supplement form, herbal teas, or tinctures.

6. **Rhodiola Rosea (Arctic Root or Golden Root)**:

- Enhances mood, energy levels, and resilience to stress.

- Supports overall mental well-being and cognitive function.

- Typically taken in supplement form.

7. **Holy Basil (Ocimum sanctum)**:

   - Adaptogenic herb that helps the body adapt to stress and reduces symptoms of anxiety and depression.

   - Improves mood and supports overall emotional balance.

   - Consumed as a tea, tincture, or added to culinary dishes.

8. **Ashwagandha (Withania somnifera)**:

   - Reduces stress and anxiety, promoting a sense of calmness and relaxation.

   - Improves mood and supports adrenal health.

   - Available in supplement form or as a powder for use in beverages or cooking.

9. **Kava Kava (Piper methysticum)**:

   - Acts as a natural sedative and anxiolytic, promoting relaxation and reducing symptoms of anxiety and stress.

   - Improves mood and promotes a sense of euphoria.

   - Typically consumed as a tea or tincture, although caution is advised due to potential liver toxicity with prolonged use.

10. **Ginseng (Panax ginseng or Panax quinquefolius)**:

   - Adaptogenic herb that helps the body adapt to stress and improves energy levels and mood.

   - Enhances cognitive function and mental clarity.

   - Consumed as a supplement or brewed into teas.

These herbs can be used individually or in combination to create herbal blends that support mood enhancement and emotional well-being. It's important to consult with a healthcare professional before adding herbal supplements to your routine, especially if you have any underlying health conditions or are taking medications.

C. Herbal Support for Sleep and Relaxation

1. **Valerian Root (Valeriana officinalis)**:

   - Acts as a natural sedative, promoting relaxation and improving sleep quality.

   - Reduces the time it takes to fall asleep and may enhance sleep duration.

   - Often consumed as a tea, tincture, or in supplement form.

2. **Lavender (Lavandula angustifolia)**:

- Calms the nervous system and reduces anxiety and stress, promoting relaxation.

   - Improves sleep quality and may alleviate insomnia symptoms.

   - Used in aromatherapy, herbal teas, and bath products.

3. **Chamomile (Matricaria chamomilla)**:

   - Contains apigenin, a compound with sedative properties that induces relaxation and improves sleep.

   - Reduces anxiety and promotes better sleep quality.

   - Consumed as a tea, tincture, or added to bathwater.

4. **Passionflower (Passiflora incarnata)**:

   - Acts as a mild sedative and anxiolytic, reducing symptoms of anxiety and promoting relaxation.

   - Improves sleep quality and may help alleviate insomnia.

   - Available in supplement form, herbal teas, or tinctures.

5. **Lemon Balm (Melissa officinalis)**:

   - Relieves stress and anxiety, promoting a sense of calmness and relaxation.

   - Enhances sleep quality and may reduce symptoms of insomnia.

- Consumed as a tea, tincture, or added to culinary dishes.

6. **California Poppy (Eschscholzia californica)**:

   - Contains compounds that induce relaxation and improve sleep quality.

   - Acts as a mild sedative and analgesic, reducing anxiety and promoting restful sleep.

   - Typically consumed as a tincture or in supplement form.

7. **Hops (Humulus lupulus)**:

   - Contains sedative compounds that promote relaxation and improve sleep quality.

   - Reduces anxiety and may alleviate symptoms of insomnia.

   - Often used in combination with other herbs in teas or tinctures.

8. **Ashwagandha (Withania somnifera)**:

   - Reduces stress and anxiety, promoting relaxation and improving sleep quality.

   - Supports adrenal health and helps the body adapt to stress.

   - Available in supplement form or as a powder for use in beverages or cooking.

9. **Skullcap (Scutellaria lateriflora)**:

   - Acts as a mild sedative and nervine, calming the nervous system and promoting relaxation.

   - Improves sleep quality and may alleviate insomnia symptoms.

   - Consumed as a tea, tincture, or in supplement form.

10. **Magnolia Bark (Magnolia officinalis)**:

   - Contains compounds that reduce anxiety and promote relaxation, improving sleep quality.

   - Acts as a mild sedative and anxiolytic, enhancing GABAergic neurotransmission.

   - Typically consumed as a supplement or in herbal teas.

These herbs can be used individually or in combination to create herbal blends that support sleep and relaxation. It's important to consult with a healthcare professional before adding herbal supplements to your routine, especially if you have any underlying health conditions or are taking medications.

IX. Herbal Medicine for Long-Term Health and Prevention

A. Herbal Tonics for Vitality and Longevity

Certainly! Here's a comprehensive list of herbal tonics for vitality and longevity, presented with bullets and numbers:

1. **Ashwagandha (Withania somnifera)**:

   - Adaptogenic herb that supports energy levels and vitality.

   - Helps reduce stress and fatigue, promoting overall well-being.

   - Available in supplement form or as a powder for use in beverages or cooking.

2. **Rhodiola Rosea (Arctic Root or Golden Root)**:

   - Enhances physical and mental performance, increasing stamina and resilience to stress.

   - Improves energy levels and supports adrenal health.

   - Typically taken in supplement form.

3. **Panax Ginseng (Asian Ginseng)**:

   - Adaptogenic herb that boosts energy, vitality, and longevity.

   - Improves cognitive function and physical endurance.

   - Available in supplement form or as a tea.

4. **Holy Basil (Ocimum sanctum)**:

   - Adaptogenic herb that increases energy levels and reduces stress.

   - Supports adrenal health and overall vitality.

   - Consumed as a tea, tincture, or added to culinary dishes.

5. **Schisandra Berry (Schisandra chinensis)**:

   - Adaptogenic herb that enhances endurance, mental clarity, and longevity.

   - Increases resistance to stress and fatigue.

   - Consumed as a tea, tincture, or in supplement form.

6. **Reishi Mushroom (Ganoderma lucidum)**:

   - Adaptogenic mushroom that supports immune function and increases vitality.

   - Enhances energy levels and reduces fatigue.

   - Available in supplement form or as a tea.

7. **Maca Root (Lepidium meyenii)**:

   - Energizing herb that increases stamina, libido, and overall vitality.

   - Helps reduce fatigue and improve mood.

- Available in powder form for use in smoothies, beverages, or cooking.

8. **Astragalus Root (Astragalus membranaceus)**:

   - Adaptogenic herb that strengthens the immune system and increases vitality.

   - Supports physical endurance and reduces fatigue.

   - Consumed as a tea, tincture, or in supplement form.

9. **Cordyceps Mushroom (Cordyceps sinensis)**:

   - Energizing mushroom that enhances physical performance and vitality.

   - Improves endurance, stamina, and oxygen utilization.

   - Available in supplement form or as a tea.

10. **Eleuthero Root (Siberian Ginseng)**:

   - Adaptogenic herb that increases energy levels and resilience to stress.

   - Supports physical endurance and mental clarity.

   - Typically consumed as a tea or in supplement form.

These herbal tonics can be used individually or in combination to support vitality, energy, and overall longevity. It's important to consult with a healthcare professional before adding herbal supplements to your routine, especially if you have any underlying health conditions or are taking medications.

B. Disease Prevention with Herbal Medicine

Disease prevention with herbal medicine involves using natural remedies to support the body's immune system, reduce inflammation, and address underlying health issues. Here's a comprehensive guide to disease prevention with herbal medicine:

1. **Boosting Immune Function**:

   - Echinacea: Enhances immune response and helps prevent colds and flu.

   - Astragalus: Supports immune function and helps prevent respiratory infections.

   - Elderberry: Rich in antioxidants and helps prevent viral infections like the flu.

   - Garlic: Boosts the immune system and has antimicrobial properties.

2. **Reducing Inflammation**:

   - Turmeric: Contains curcumin, a potent anti-inflammatory compound.

- Ginger: Helps reduce inflammation and supports digestive health.

- Boswellia: Reduces inflammation and may alleviate symptoms of arthritis.

- Green Tea: Rich in antioxidants that combat inflammation and support overall health.

3. **Supporting Cardiovascular Health**:

- Hawthorn: Supports heart health and helps prevent cardiovascular disease.

- Garlic: Lowers cholesterol and blood pressure, reducing the risk of heart disease.

- Cayenne Pepper: Improves circulation and supports cardiovascular function.

- Ginkgo Biloba: Enhances blood flow and may reduce the risk of stroke and heart disease.

4. **Promoting Digestive Health**:

- Peppermint: Relieves indigestion and supports gastrointestinal function.

- Ginger: Helps alleviate nausea and supports digestion.

- Slippery Elm: Soothes irritated mucous membranes and promotes healing in the digestive tract.

- Licorice Root: Supports digestive health and helps prevent ulcers.

5. **Maintaining Cognitive Function**:

   - Ginkgo Biloba: Improves circulation to the brain and supports cognitive function.

   - Bacopa: Enhances memory and cognitive performance.

   - Rosemary: Contains compounds that support brain health and cognitive function.

   - Ashwagandha: Reduces stress and may help prevent age-related cognitive decline.

6. **Balancing Hormones**:

   - Vitex (Chasteberry): Helps regulate hormonal balance and alleviate symptoms of PMS.

   - Dong Quai: Supports female reproductive health and balances hormones.

   - Saw Palmetto: Supports prostate health and helps balance hormones in men.

   - Maca: Adaptogenic herb that supports hormone balance and overall vitality.

7. **Antioxidant Support**:

- Green Tea: Rich in antioxidants that protect cells from oxidative damage.

- Rosehip: High in vitamin C and antioxidants that support immune function and skin health.

- Bilberry: Supports eye health and contains antioxidants that promote overall well-being.

- Amla (Indian Gooseberry): Rich in vitamin C and antioxidants that support immune function and cellular health.

8. **Detoxification**:

- Milk Thistle: Supports liver health and detoxification processes in the body.

- Dandelion Root: Supports liver function and aids in detoxification.

- Burdock Root: Cleanses the blood and supports overall detoxification.

- Nettle: Supports kidney function and helps eliminate toxins from the body.

9. **Stress Management**:

- Holy Basil: Adaptogenic herb that helps the body adapt to stress and promotes relaxation.

- Rhodiola: Reduces stress and fatigue, supporting overall well-being.

- Ashwagandha: Helps reduce stress and promotes relaxation.

  - Lemon Balm: Calms the nervous system and reduces anxiety and stress.

10. **Bone and Joint Health**:

  - Turmeric: Contains anti-inflammatory properties that help reduce joint pain and inflammation.

  - Boswellia: Supports joint health and reduces inflammation associated with arthritis.

  - Nettle Leaf: Rich in nutrients that support bone health and reduce inflammation.

  - Horsetail: High in silica, which supports bone and connective tissue health.

Incorporating these herbal remedies into a balanced lifestyle can help support overall health and well-being, reducing the risk of disease and promoting longevity. It's essential to consult with a healthcare professional before starting any herbal regimen, especially if you have existing health conditions or are taking medications.

C. Holistic Wellness Practices

Holistic wellness practices encompass various approaches that aim to promote well-being by considering the whole person—mind, body, and spirit. Here's a comprehensive guide to holistic wellness practices:

1. **Mindfulness and Meditation**:

- Practice mindfulness meditation to cultivate awareness of the present moment and reduce stress.

- Engage in guided meditation sessions to promote relaxation and mental clarity.

- Incorporate mindfulness into daily activities such as eating, walking, and breathing exercises.

2. **Yoga and Tai Chi**:

- Practice yoga or tai chi to improve flexibility, strength, and balance.

- These mind-body practices also promote relaxation, reduce stress, and enhance overall well-being.

- Attend classes or follow online tutorials to learn different poses and techniques.

3. **Nutrition and Healthy Eating**:

- Focus on whole, nutrient-dense foods such as fruits, vegetables, whole grains, lean proteins, and healthy fats.

- Limit processed foods, sugary beverages, and excessive amounts of salt and added sugars.

- Pay attention to portion sizes and practice mindful eating to fully enjoy and appreciate your meals.

4. **Physical Activity and Exercise**:

- Incorporate regular physical activity into your daily routine, such as walking, jogging, cycling, or swimming.

- Aim for at least 150 minutes of moderate-intensity exercise or 75 minutes of vigorous-intensity exercise per week.

- Find activities you enjoy to make exercise a sustainable part of your lifestyle.

5. **Stress Management**:

- Practice relaxation techniques such as deep breathing, progressive muscle relaxation, or guided imagery.

- Engage in activities that help you unwind and reduce stress, such as spending time in nature, listening to music, or practicing hobbies.

- Set boundaries, prioritize self-care, and learn to say no to excessive commitments.

6. **Quality Sleep**:

- Prioritize sleep by establishing a consistent sleep schedule and creating a relaxing bedtime routine.

- Create a sleep-friendly environment by keeping your bedroom dark, quiet, and cool.

- Avoid screens and stimulating activities before bedtime, and limit caffeine and alcohol intake in the evening.

7. **Emotional Well-being**:

   - Practice self-care activities that nurture your emotional well-being, such as journaling, spending time with loved ones, or seeking support from a therapist or counselor.

   - Cultivate gratitude and optimism by focusing on positive aspects of your life and practicing gratitude exercises.

   - Develop healthy coping mechanisms to manage stress, anxiety, and difficult emotions.

8. **Social Connections**:

   - Foster meaningful relationships with friends, family, and community members.

   - Make time for social activities and gatherings that bring joy and fulfillment.

   - Seek out support networks and participate in group activities or clubs with shared interests.

9. **Spiritual Practices**:

   - Engage in spiritual or religious practices that provide a sense of purpose, meaning, and connection.

   - Explore mindfulness-based approaches to spirituality, such as meditation, prayer, or contemplative practices.

- Connect with nature and explore the natural world as a source of inspiration and spiritual renewal.

10. **Holistic Healthcare**:

- Consider complementary and alternative therapies such as acupuncture, chiropractic care, massage therapy, or herbal medicine to support your overall health and well-being.

- Work with holistic healthcare practitioners who take an integrative approach to address your unique needs and concerns.

By integrating these holistic wellness practices into your daily life, you can enhance your overall health and well-being, promote balance and harmony, and cultivate a greater sense of vitality and vitality. Remember that everyone's journey to wellness is unique, so experiment with different approaches and find what works best for you.

X. Conclusion

Embracing Nature's Wisdom:

Throughout history, humans have turned to medicinal herbs for their healing properties, harnessing the power of nature to promote health and well-being.

A Holistic Approach to Wellness:

The use of medicinal herbs embodies a holistic approach to wellness, addressing not only physical ailments but also mental, emotional, and spiritual aspects of health.

Harnessing the Healing Power of Plants:

Medicinal herbs offer a diverse array of healing compounds, including antioxidants, anti-inflammatory agents, and immune-boosting substances, among others.

Empowering Self-Care:

Learning about medicinal herbs empowers individuals to take control of their health and well-being, offering natural alternatives to conventional medicine and promoting self-care practices.

Cultivating Connection with Nature:

Engaging with medicinal herbs fosters a deeper connection with the natural world, encouraging mindfulness, appreciation for biodiversity, and stewardship of the environment.

An Ongoing Journey of Discovery:

The study of medicinal herbs is an ongoing journey of discovery, as researchers uncover new therapeutic properties and traditional wisdom is passed down through generations.

Integration with Conventional Medicine:

Integrating medicinal herbs with conventional medicine offers a comprehensive approach to health care, combining the strengths of both systems to optimize patient outcomes.

Respect for Traditional Wisdom:

Honoring traditional wisdom and cultural practices surrounding medicinal herbs ensures the preservation of valuable knowledge and promotes cultural diversity in healing traditions.

Promoting Sustainable Practices:

Sustainable harvesting and cultivation practices are essential to ensure the availability of medicinal herbs for future generations, emphasizing the importance of ethical sourcing and conservation efforts.

Empowering Healing and Wholeness:

In conclusion, The Complete Guide to Medicinal Herbs serves as a comprehensive resource for harnessing nature's healing power, empowering individuals to embrace holistic wellness and cultivate a deeper connection with the natural world for healing and wholeness.

In summary, The Complete Guide to Medicinal Herbs offers a wealth of information and resources for individuals interested in exploring the healing potential of medicinal herbs. By embracing nature's wisdom, cultivating a holistic approach to wellness, and integrating medicinal herbs into our lives, we can promote health, vitality, and harmony with the natural world.

A. Embracing the Power of Medicinal Herbs

In today's fast-paced world, where stress, pollution, and processed foods are ubiquitous, it's no wonder that many people are seeking natural remedies to support their health and well-being. One such remedy that has stood the test of time is medicinal herbs. Embracing the power of medicinal herbs offers not just relief from symptoms but also a path to holistic wellness that encompasses the mind, body, and spirit.

Ancient Wisdom Rediscovered:

The use of medicinal herbs dates back thousands of years, with cultures around the world incorporating plants into their healing practices. From Ayurveda in India to Traditional Chinese Medicine to Native American herbalism, ancient wisdom has long recognized the therapeutic properties of herbs.

Harnessing Nature's Pharmacy:

Medicinal herbs are nature's pharmacy, containing a vast array of bioactive compounds that can have profound effects on our health. From anti-inflammatory and antioxidant properties to immune-boosting and mood-enhancing effects, herbs offer a holistic approach to healing.

Promoting Holistic Healing:

Unlike conventional medicine, which often focuses solely on treating symptoms, medicinal herbs address the root cause of illness by promoting balance and harmony within the body. By supporting the body's innate ability to heal itself, herbs offer a holistic approach to healing that encompasses physical, emotional, mental, and spiritual well-being.

Supporting Self-Care Practices:

One of the most empowering aspects of medicinal herbs is that they put the power of healing back into the hands of the individual. By incorporating herbs into our daily routines, we can take proactive steps to support our health and prevent illness. Whether it's brewing a cup of herbal tea, adding herbs to our meals, or using herbal remedies for common ailments, herbs offer simple yet effective ways to practice self-care.

Natural Remedies for Modern Ailments:

In an era of pharmaceuticals and synthetic treatments, medicinal herbs offer a gentler, more sustainable approach to health care. Whether it's using ginger to ease digestive discomfort, lavender to promote relaxation, or echinacea to support the immune system, herbs provide natural alternatives for addressing a wide range of health concerns.

Cultivating Connection with Nature:

Embracing medicinal herbs is not just about healing the body; it's also about fostering a deeper connection with the natural world. By learning about herbs, growing them in our gardens, and harvesting them sustainably, we can cultivate a sense of reverence for the plants that nourish and sustain us.

Honoring Traditional Knowledge:

In embracing the power of medicinal herbs, we also honor the wisdom of our ancestors and indigenous cultures. By learning from traditional healers and herbalists, we can gain valuable insights into the therapeutic properties of plants and the importance of living in harmony with nature.

Empowering Wellness Choices:

By embracing medicinal herbs, we empower ourselves to make informed choices about our health. Whether we choose to use herbs as complementary therapies alongside conventional medicine or as standalone treatments, herbs offer us a wealth of options for supporting our well-being.

Promoting Sustainability and Conservation:

As we embrace the power of medicinal herbs, it's essential to do so responsibly. By supporting ethical harvesting practices, promoting sustainable cultivation methods, and protecting endangered plant species, we can ensure that future generations will continue to benefit from the healing power of herbs.

Embracing a Path to Wholeness:

Ultimately, embracing the power of medicinal herbs is about embracing a path to wholeness. It's about recognizing that true wellness encompasses not just the absence of disease but also a state of balance, vitality, and harmony within ourselves and the world around us.

In conclusion, embracing the power of medicinal herbs is a journey— one that offers us not just relief from symptoms but also a deeper connection with ourselves, with nature, and with the wisdom of our ancestors. It's a journey that invites us to reclaim our health, empower ourselves, and embrace a holistic approach to wellness that honors the intricate interconnectedness of all living beings. So let us embrace the power of medicinal herbs and embark on this journey to holistic wellness together.

B. The Future of Herbal Medicine

As we stand on the cusp of a new era in healthcare, the future of herbal medicine shines brightly as a beacon of hope and healing. In a world increasingly plagued by chronic diseases, antibiotic resistance, and environmental degradation, the resurgence of interest in herbal medicine offers a promising path forward—one that integrates ancient wisdom with modern science to promote health and well-being for generations to come.

1. **Integrating Traditional Knowledge with Modern Science**:

   - The future of herbal medicine lies in bridging the gap between traditional knowledge and modern scientific research. By combining the wisdom of ancient healing traditions with the rigors of modern scientific inquiry, we can unlock the full potential of medicinal plants and their therapeutic compounds.

2. **Harnessing the Power of Plant-Based Medicine**:

   - As the shortcomings of conventional pharmaceuticals become increasingly apparent, there is growing interest in plant-based alternatives. Herbal medicine offers a treasure trove of botanical remedies that can address a wide range of health conditions, from chronic pain and inflammation to mental health disorders and immune system support.

3. **Personalized Medicine and Individualized Care**:

   - One of the most exciting developments in the future of herbal medicine is the shift towards personalized medicine and individualized care. By recognizing that each person is unique and may respond differently to herbal treatments, practitioners can tailor remedies to meet the specific needs of each patient, leading to more effective and personalized healthcare.

4. **Advancements in Herbal Formulations and Delivery Methods**:

   - With advances in technology and innovation, herbal medicine is undergoing a renaissance in formulation and delivery methods. From standardized herbal extracts and nanoencapsulation techniques to novel delivery systems such as transdermal patches and inhalers, the future of herbal medicine holds promise for greater efficacy, bioavailability, and patient compliance.

5. **Cultivating Sustainability and Environmental Stewardship**:

   - As interest in herbal medicine continues to grow, so too does the need for sustainable harvesting and cultivation practices. The future of herbal medicine depends on our ability to protect and preserve medicinal plant species and their habitats, ensuring their availability for future generations.

6. **Empowering Self-Care and Preventive Healthcare**:

   - Herbal medicine empowers individuals to take an active role in their own health and well-being. By promoting self-care practices and preventive healthcare strategies, herbal medicine can help reduce the burden of chronic disease and improve overall quality of life.

7. **Integration with Conventional Healthcare Systems**:

   - The future of herbal medicine lies in its integration with conventional healthcare systems. As more research is conducted and evidence-based practices are established, herbal medicine will continue to gain recognition and acceptance within mainstream healthcare, offering complementary and alternative options for patients.

8. **Cultivating Collaboration and Cross-Cultural Exchange**:

- In an increasingly interconnected world, the future of herbal medicine depends on collaboration and cross-cultural exchange. By sharing knowledge, resources, and best practices across diverse cultures and traditions, we can enrich our understanding of herbal medicine and promote global health and well-being.

In conclusion, the future of herbal medicine is bright and full of promise. By embracing tradition in modern healthcare, we can harness the healing power of medicinal plants to address the complex health challenges of our time. From integrating traditional knowledge with modern science to promoting sustainability and environmental stewardship, herbal medicine offers a holistic and sustainable approach to health and healing—one that honors the wisdom of the past while paving the way for a healthier future for all.

www.ingramcontent.com/pod-product-compliance
Lightning Source LLC
Chambersburg PA
CBHW031413250726

48656CB00002B/663